WEIGHT LOSS WITH DR SEBI APPROACH

• • • Food and health via Dr Sebi approach.

(Brenda S. Hardin)

Table of Contents

Dedication

I dedicate this book to you for sacrificing your time and resources in pursuit of knowledge towards a healthier lifestyle.

INTRODUCTION

Excess weight gain has been implicated as the cause of many medical diseases, some of which include hypertension, diabetes, heart diseases, gout, sleep apnea osteoarthritis, to mention but a few. Not to mention the social ostracization many overweight people experience within the society, and this has been a cause of concern. The truth is most of the abundance of fat people tend to accumulate from eating unhealthy diets or indulging in unhealthy lifestyles. Several studies have shown that people who live a healthy lifestyle and places inhibition on the food they eat have less fat deposit than people who doesn't. This book will take you through healthy diets that you can include in your food menu and those classes of food you need to cut out or reduce to achieve the result you want. Also, you get to learn about those habits you need to stop and those daily routines you need to inculcate in your fight against excess weight. Enjoy!

CHAPTER ONE

WHO DR SEBI WAS

The name Dr. Sebi was an alias for a man named Alfredo Darrignton Bowman. He was a Honduran herbalist (i.e., orthodox medicine practitioner) and a self-proclaimed healer who claimed to have developed a unique approach and methodology to the healing of a human body irrespective of the disease with the sole use of herbs and food supplements. He was known to practice his form of medicine in the United States between the late 20th and early 21st century. He was recorded to be born on 26th of November, 1933 to Clifford Bowman and Violet Francis Bowman in Illanga, Honduras, and died 6th of August 2016 in La Ceiba, Honduras. He was married to Patsy Bowman and Maha Bowman. He was survived by 17 children. Dr Sebi is of the firm belief that diseases thrive in an acidic environment and as a result of the mucous build-up in a part of the body and mostly recommended alkaline diet, which is usually plant-based. He claims that cell rejuvenation occurs by the elimination of toxic was which happen when the body is being alkalized. He claims that the preference of certain foods and avoidance of some other foods could help to detoxify the body and achieve the state of health necessary to reduce the risk and effects of diseases. Most of this diet has been known to help in weight reduction as they reduce the calorie intake, thereby encouraging the body to use the stored fat cells for the needed energy. They also boost body metabolism, thereby enhancing weight loss.

CHAPTER TWO

WEIGHT GAIN

Weight gain is the addition of pound to body mass, which often occurs as a result of overeating or lack of physical activity. Studies have shown that obesity is one of the biggest health problems in the world. Though it usually ensues as a result of eating habits and lifestyles, some people are at a disadvantage as they are genetically predisposed to weight gain. Some factors contribute to weight gain.

1. Genetics: The fact is obesity has a strong genetic component and can easily be inherited from parents. This does not necessarily mean obesity is predetermined in people as what you eat also contributes greatly to what gene is expressed and what gene is not.

2. Processed food: Over time, processed food has become the food of choice for many people. This food is designed to be cheap, last long o the shelf, and they taste so good that they become irresistible. Not to talk of the fact that many of these foods come already made, which takes off the stress of having to prepare them.

These factors promote overeating. This, in addition to the high-calorie content, most processed food carries contributes to weight gain.

3. Insulin: This is the hormone production by the pancreas. It helps the body to use glucose from carbohydrates as energy, and it also helps to store glucose as glycogen. Alongside this, insulin also enhances the ability of fat cells to store more fat in the body by inhibiting the breakdown of fat cells. It tells the body to stop burning fat and to absorb more fatty acids, which contributes a great deal to an increase in body fat.

4. Medications: Certain medications like antipsychotics, antidepressants, and diabetes medication have been known to have weight has their side effect. They alter the function of the body and brain, thereby reducing the body's metabolic rate and increasing appetite.

5. Leptin resistance: Leptin is a hormone that is produced by the fat cells of the body. It is called appetite-reducing hormone as it helps to put human appetite in check. It helps to reduce hunger and increase energy expenditure in the body. Though leptin suppresses appetite when it is slightly raised, it performs the

opposite when it is too high. Most obese people tend to have available leptin in their bodies. Which means there is an indicator telling their brain how much fat it has stored.

6. Sugar: Sugar is found in virtually every diet these days. It tends to change the hormone and biochemistry of the body when taken in excess, thereby making its contribution to weight gain. Excess sugar intake has been known to cause a high insulin level in the body. Instead of bringing satiety, most sugar content increases craving, thereby contributing to increased energy storage and obesity.

7. Stress: The body secrets a hormone called cortisol when we are stressed. This hormone is, at times, referred to as stress hormone. It increases appetite and sugar cravings because these hormones cause an increase in insulin level in the body, which tends to make people prefer comfort food high in sugar and fat when they are stressed. Stress also dials own the level leptin, which is supposed to give a feeling of fullness or satiety.

WHAT DR SEBI SAID ABOUT WEIGHT LOSS

Dr. Sebi's diet therapy promotes an unprocessed plant-based diet. Compared to the western diet, people who follow a plant-based diet have lower rates of obesity. A 12-month study that was performed in this regard shows that people who follow an unlimited whole food, low fat, plant-based diet lose a significant amount of weight than people who didn't follow the diet. Dr. Sebi's diet involves eating vegetables, fruits, grains, nuts and seeds, herbal teas, natural sweeteners, and spices. This diet contributes greatly to weight loss and appetite control, thereby helping to put the body fat in check. They are packed with fibers, which helps to stay full for a more extended period and, in turn, reduces the need to keep getting stuffed with food. Dr. Sebi's diet therapy is deficient in fat and refined grains. It contains no cholesterol, no processed sugar, and no alcohol, all of which contribute significantly to weight gain.

CHAPTER THREE

FOOD THAT

CONTRIBUTES TO

WEIGHT LOSS

Apart from the need to stay in shape and good health, excess weight gain is often seen as off-putting in our society. Most overweight people tend to have low self-esteem because of the constant stigmatization and inability to fit appropriately within the society. Several discriminatory behaviors are most times targeted at obese people. Social media has offered no help in this aspect also as most ideal beauty portrayed by social media are people who are of a certain weight, looks, and height, and this has to heighten social anxiety amidst people who are overweight. The good news is the weight doesn't have to remain; there is something that can be done. Several foods have been known to contribute to weight loss and also help to put the habits that support weight gain in check.

HIGH PROTEIN DIET

A high protein diet includes a large quantity of protein and only a small quantity of carbohydrates. Food that is rich in protein helps a person to feel full, thereby reducing the need for more calorie intake. A high protein diet has been known to have an impressive impact on the appetite, the body's metabolic rate, and the body's composition. Protein diets produce certain hormones on the body that helps to feel full and satisfied. It also reduces the production of the hormone ghrelin, which is also known as the hunger hormone. All these factors combined automatically leads to a natural reduction in food intake. High protein diet also increases the number of calories you burn most, especially when combined with exercise, as this helps to build lean muscle in the body, and they are renowned for their ability to burn excess calories in the body throughout the day. Studies have shown that it does this by boosting the metabolic rate by about a whopping 20-35%. This also promotes weight and fat loss. Daily intake of about 1.2-1.6 grams per kilogram of your weigh of a high protein diet can help to promote fat loss.

Some excellent protein choices include; eggs, lean beef, beans, shrimp, nuts and seeds, fish, lentils, oats, dairy products, vegetables, broccoli, cauliflower, cabbage, chicken breast, tuna, tempeh, spirulina, legumes, guava, peas, almonds, avocado, chia seeds, halibut, asparagus, Brussels sprouts, watercress, spelled, pistachios, etc.

LOW-CALORIE DIET

Contrary to many people's opinions, a low-calorie diet does not mean low on nutrients. It just means feeding your body with healthy foods that support your health and enhances weight loss. Low-calorie diets are a diet that reduces calorie intake to about 1200-1600 per day for men and 1000-1200 per day for women. Some people go on a very low-calorie diet, consuming only about 800 calories per day. But for effective weight loss without adverse effects, a low-calorie diet is advised against a deficient calorie diet. This is because a less extreme diet is very easier to adhere to, and they tend to interrupt daily activities less. Though most low-calorie diets leave you feeling hungry and unfulfilled between meals, a good combination with a high protein diet will help to resolve the issue, and there is some low-calorie diet that can give you the feeling of fullness and satiety that you desire. By eating a low-calorie diet, you create a calorie deficit that can ultimately lead to weight loss. The logic with a low-calorie diet is when you eat less calories than your body burns, the body results in burning the fat store of the body to make up for the calorie shortfall.

Some good examples include oat, berries, eggs, chia seeds, cottage cheese, potatoes, lean meat, legumes, watermelon, tomatoes, walnut, soup, shakes, celery, arugula, radish, cucumber, grapefruits, wheat bran, mussels, lentils, etc.

WATER

Drinking water has been known to help boost metabolism, and this, in turn, helps to burn excess fat in the body. It is also known to be actively involved in cleaning the body of waste and act as an appetite suppressant. Studies have shown that drinking more water helps the body to stop retaining water, leading to a significant drop in the extra pound gotten from water weight. It is advised that water is taken before meals. Because it is an appetite suppressant, it will reduce the amount of food you eat. The average reduction in calories in intake measures up to 75 calories when water is taken before a meal. You can only imagine how many calories you will lose per day, week, month, or year if you decide to start taking water before each meal. Studies have shown that by replacing calorie-filled drinks with water, you tend to lose more weight. If you think water tastes boring, you can add lemon to the water has this has a good track record in helping to enhance weight loss. It is better to drink this water cold as the body has to work harder to warm the water up, thereby boosting metabolism. For people who are strong and healthy enough, water fasting is also advised. This means the intake of water alone without food for a while because the body does not have calories to feed on. It results in burning the fat deposit in the body to provide the body with energy.

FIBRE

There are two types of fibre, soluble fibre, and insoluble fibre. Insoluble

fibre does not mix with water. It acts
as a bulking agent to help form stools.
Soluble water, on the other hand,
mixes with water to form a viscous
gel-like substance, which slows down
how fast the stomach releases food
into the gut and gives a feeling of
fullness, thereby reducing the need for
more food intake. Fibres are known to
feed friendly bacteria in the gut.
These bacteria contribute significantly
to various aspects of the health of
which weight management is one.
Fibres make the stomach full, thereby
stimulating the centre in the brain that
tells us to stop eating. Besides, fibres
are more slowly digested than other
carbohydrates, which means food

stays in your stomach for a longer period of time, and you don't feel the need to eat often.

Some examples include beans, flax seeds, legumes, asparagus, Brussels sprouts, oats, berries, barley, brown rice, bran, spinach, carrots, green beans, banana, prunes, apple, peanuts, squash, guava, figs, kiwi, beets, etc.

PLANT-BASED DIET

Most plant-based diets have low-calorie density; by taking them, you will be ingesting food that is low in calories and still gives you the feeling of fullness that you desire. The fact is natural; unprocessed food is loaded with fibre and water, which has discussed above contributes significantly to weight loss. Though some people relate plant-based diets to vegan foods, the main idea is to make a plant-based diet the central part of your meals. The emphasis of plant-based diets is on fruits, vegetables, beans, nuts, etc. Though seafood, meat, egg, and dairy products do not necessarily have to be off-limits, you might need to cut back on your intake of them. Proper adherence to a plant-based diet will help you maintain a healthy weight.

LOW-FAT DIET

Most of the excess weight of the body comes from the abundance of fat deposits that are gotten from consumption of calories the body doesn't need and also from the consumption of unhealthy food products. There are about four different types of fats they include saturated fats, monounsaturated fats, polyunsaturated fats, and Trans-fat. Saturated fats contain excess calories. They are found in meat, hotdogs, bacon, sausages, which add those additional fats the body doesn't need. Monounsaturated fats contribute greatly to weight loss as they contain less calories. They support healthy energy levels in the body. They are found in avocado, olives and olive oil, macadamia nuts. Polyunsaturated fat includes omega 3 and omega 6, which are good for the heart and healthy for the body. They are found in salmon, flaxseed, coconut oil, etc. the trans-fats are the worst kind of fat. This is because they are the product of the hydrogenation of healthy oils, which makes it unhealthy for the body. By taking a low-fat diet, you cut down on the great number of calories that are found in fat diets. Studies have shown that the standard low-fat diet lowers your calorie intake by about 30% of the usual daily fat intake. Fats contain about 9 calories per gram, which is quite high compared to 4 calories per gram contained in protein. It is advised to eat boiled or baked foods instead of fried foods for a low-fat diet, chicken and turkey should be peeled skinless before they are eaten, cut down on fatty diaries it is better to go for skimmed milk, low fat yoghurt, and cheese. Opt for leafy greens and fruits. Mushroom, garlic, white fish, egg whites, sweet potatoes contain low fat.

DASH DIET

DASH simply means Dietary Approach to Stop Hypertension (DASH). DASH diet is usually used for the prevention and treatment of hypertension. The emphasis and focus of dash diet are on fruits, vegetables, whole grains, nuts, low-fat dairy, legumes and lean meats which is the more reason why it is recommended for people who are trying to lose weight as it prevents the intake of excess calories that adds to the body's fat deposit. By taking the dash diet, there have been positive reports of who lose weight as they ingest less unhealthy fats and low sugar content. One of the reasons why DASH diet is the weight loss choice for many people is because it is more flexible than other diet plans. The sad news is a lot of people have refused to choose the dash diet for weight control because of some misconceptions they have. Some of this misconception includes: dash diet is only for people with hypertension, it only focuses on low sodium and no salt intake, it is unapproachable and many other ones. But the truth is the health benefit of taking dash diets goes beyond weight loss, and it is worth a try. Most studies have shown that DASH dieting is about sustainability. This means the dietary control is focused on the diet you can maintain and keep up with.

PALEO DIET

Paleo diet obtained its name from the fact that it contains food in the past that could only be obtained by hunting and gathering. These foods are known to be heavy on protein and low in carbs. It focuses on avoiding processed food that contains high fat and sodium. It encourages healthy whole foods. With the paleo diet, you eat food that fills you up and make you feel less hungry throughout the day, thereby reducing unnecessary intake of additional calories. It also helps to reduce appetite and cut down on the rate at which we eat. Though the paleo diet might be a little difficult to follow because of its high restrictions. The benefits are great as it encourages the intake of fruits, veggies, fish, poultry, nuts, seeds, meats, healthy fats, etc.

CHAPTER FOUR

ROUTINES THAT HELPS

SHED WEIGHT

The importance of watching what you eat in the fight against excess weight cannot be overemphasized. While following all the dietary changes that were mentioned above, there is a need to include routines that will hasten your result, support your health, and help to keep you in shape. Many times, people tend just to follow the food regimen, and they ignore those daily routines that tend to make them add weight. Some of this habit include inadequate or excess sleep, skipping meals, eating too quickly, watching too much television, eating off large plates, drinking too little water, eating when emotional, sitting too long, too little protein or fibres, having irregular meal times and many other habits. There are some daily routines that you can imbibe that will help in this fight against weight gain

INTERMITTENT FASTING

Intermittent fasting is also known as intermittent energy restriction that involves meal timing schedules between a voluntary fasting period and a non-fasting period. Intermittent fasting has a good track record of contributing weight loss and improving metabolic health. There are three methods of intermittent fasting. There is alternate day fasting, the periodic fasting, and the time-restricted feeding. Time-restricted feeding is the most common and most selected option as it is more convenient and adaptable. In this type of alternate fasting method, the feeding period is restricted to a certain number of hours per day, the 16 fasting hours followed by 8 non-fasting hours 16:8 cycle. In this cycle, you fast for 16 hours then eat for the next 8 hours. The 16 hours fasting is preferably done overnight, after which the first meal of the day is taken around 10 or 11 am. This period of feeding continues for the next 8 hours until about 6 pm or 7 pm; then the fasting cycle starts again. During this fasting period, you are allowed to take water, which you can mix with lemon to make it taste more interesting. It is important that you watch what you eat in this non-fasting period. Intermittent fasting is not a justifiable reason to eat whatever you want. This will only make you add the calories you lost during the fasting period. You need to follow the food regimen that has been above to have an adequate result. Intermittent fasting cuts the calorie intake per day, and the body makes up for this by getting the necessary energy from the fast deposit of the body.

SLEEP

To be considered to have had enough sleep, you must have slept at least 7 hours a day. This is because sleep deprivation makes people feel hungrier, has less satisfaction after meals, and makes them feel too weak for any exercise. Besides, it has already been discussed that leptin is a hormone that brings about satiety and fullness, and ghrelin is a hormone that stimulates hunger. Sleep deprivation reduces the level of leptin that is being released in the body and increases the level of ghrelin. This causes you to feel hungrier and less satisfied. Cortisol is another hormone also produced in high quantity as a result of inadequate sleep. Cortisol will not only make you want to eat more food, but it will also inhibit the breakdown of fat for energy and cause the body to breakdown the body's muscle for energy, which is unhealthy. The fact is when people are staying awake; they try to lean on heavy coffee and late-night snacking to keep them going. This will increase their carb intake, which we are ultimately trying to avoid while losing weight. Studies have shown that when dieters cut back on sleep, the weight they lost from fat drops by about 55% even when they maintain the same level of calories they used before the sleep deprivation. Sleep deprivation dulls the activity of the frontal lobe of the brain; this lobe is in charge of decision making and self-control. More so, the reward centre of the brain is more stimulated by food when you deprive yourself of adequate sleep. To get a positive result in your weight loss regimen, sufficient sleep is a must observe.

EXERCISES

To lose more weight, you need to burn more weight than you consume, and exercise helps to achieve this. Aerobic exercise, also known as cardio, is the major type of exercise that helps in weight loss as it is effective in burning calories. It includes walking, cycling, running, swimming, yoga, weight training, pilates. Exercises increase body metabolism; when this is combined with a healthy diet, it becomes more effective in helping to lose weight. For many people, incorporating the time for exercise into their schedule is the main issue. It doesn't have to be difficult. You can decide to take your bike or walk while running errands, use the stairs instead of opting for the convenience of the elevator, park further away from your destination, and walk the remaining distance.

Work yoga and swimming into your leisure time, and you will be able to engage in the exercises needed for weight loss.

SUN

The thought of losing weight through the help of sunlight sounds funny. Studies have shown that fat cells are sensitive to sunlight, especially the blue light emitted by the sun. So that early morning sun might just be the spice you need to add to your weight gain regimen. The fat cells beneath our skin shrink on exposure to sunlight, and less exposure to sunlight causes more fat to be stored in the cell. This is the body's way of insulating the body for warmth since there is little or no exposure to an external source of warmth. Additional weight gain is usually noticed during the winter holidays and for people that live and work in conditions where there is little or no exposure to any external source of warmth. Many people's daily routine involves moving from their air-conditioned house to their air-conditioned cars, air-conditioned office, and back to the house again. This does not enhance weight loss. It is imperative that you know this does not invite you to sit in the sun as too much sun rays can be adverse on the skin and your health. But the early morning sun on your way to work or the late evening sun while running errands might be helpful. There are days when the sunlight is so lenient you can choose these days to take a walk around your neighborhood.

ALCOHOL

There are several misconceptions that alcohol helps to burn excess fat in the body. This might be due to the hot sensation many people feel when they take this hard drink, they seem to believe that hotness also goes into the fat deposit of the body. Studies have shown that alcohol acts on the contrary and is an enemy you need to avoid in this fight against excess weight. Alcoholic drinks are filled with empty calories, which means they supply the body with excess calories with little or no nutrients. When alcohol is consumed, the body tends to burn its calorie as a fuel source first before using anything else which means the excess glucose and lipids ends up getting stored as fat instead on being used as a source of energy. Alcoholic drinks have an adverse effect on the liver, which plays an important role in the metabolism of fat. Liver diseases will affect fats, carbohydrates, and protein metabolism, which ultimately leads to the accumulation of excess fat in the body. In addition, alcohol lowers inhibition and self-control; this makes you find yourself doing things you will not usually do or do not want to do while under the influence of alcohol. It also lowers the levels of some sex hormones like testosterone, which is renowned for its ability to enhance metabolism, lose excess weight, and gain lean muscle.

Thank you for making it through to the end of this book. I hope it has been informative and helpful enough to supply you with the tools you need to win this fight. The truth is it is not only about reading these books; it is about putting it to practice. You don't have to choose all the regimens and methods provided in this book; you just have to study them carefully and choose one that works for you and one you can quickly adapt to. Consistency is a very important key, so choosing a regimen, you will be able to keep up with is the best way to go. I wish you the best of luck as you swing to action.